# Infertility Can SUCK LESS!

## How to Take Control & Ownership of Your Infertility Struggles

By
Pradeepa Narayanaswamy

Dear Elyse,
  Thank you for your love &
support. I am grateful for
your friendship. Together we
can help infertility suck less!
    With lots of love,

*Pready*

Infertility Can SUCK LESS! How to take control and ownership of your fertility struggles

Published in the United States by BCG Publishing, 2020.

www.BCGPublishing.com

# Disclaimer

The following viewpoints in this book are those of Pradeepa Narayanaswamy. These views are based on her personal experience with infertility for over twelve years and eleven years as a professional coach helping others and now four years as a fertility coach.

The intention of this book is to share her story with infertility and what she learned through this journey. Her hope is that this book will inspire people to take action and own their fertility journey instead of being a victim.

All attempts have been made to verify the information provided by this publication. Neither the author nor the publisher assumes any responsibility for errors, omissions, or contrary interpretations of the subject matter herein.

This book is for entertainment purposes only. The views expressed are those of the author alone and should not be taken as expert instructions or commands. The reader is responsible for his or her future action. This book makes absolutely no guarantee of having a baby. However, by following the tips and techniques that are listed in this book, you have a high chance of success in making your infertility suck less!

Neither the author nor the publisher assumes any responsibility or liability on behalf of the purchaser or reader of these materials. The views expressed are based on her personal experiences within the corporate world, education, and everyday life.

This book is dedicated to my lovely mother, Krishnaveni, my late father, Narayanaswamy, my dear husband, Sai, and my sweet son, Kartik. Without their love and support I would not be here today.

I am dedicating this to all my dear friends and family who have cheered, supported, and motivated me to continue moving forward in my fertility coaching journey!

I am also dedicating this book to all my clients whom I had the privilege to coach and support in their fertility journey! I am super proud of each and every one as you took the coaching to your heart and took control and ownership of your infertility struggles and turned them around for good.

# Table of Contents

# Invitation to Join My Facebook Support Group

My personal experience as a member for twelve years with many online and in-person support groups felt like a pity party to me. I rarely felt inspired or motivated. I often found myself desperately seeking medical information from people in the group who were not trained medical doctors or specialists. Now, having seen the light at the end of the tunnel with my fertility struggles, I created this online Facebook support group called NOT YOUR TYPICAL INFERTILITY SUPPORT GROUP that is inviting, inspiring, uplifting, positive! Here is what the group stands for.

# Not Your Typical Fertility Support Group Manifesto

- This is a place that offers positive, humorous and uplifting messages for those going through the turmoil of life with infertility.
- This will be a place to share our common experiences with infertility.
- This will be a place where your safety guards can come down and you can be yourself.
- This is a place where you are respected as a human being rather than a fertility treatment/age category.
- This is a place where everyone can offer their opinion without being judged irrespective of your struggles, decisions and perspectives.
- This is a place where you have friends you haven't met yet who are willing to offer you a shoulder to cry on and an amazing hug!
- This is a place for you to unwind with your favorite beverage at the end of a stressful day.
- This is a place where you can continuously rely on a strong support structure outside of your partner.
- This is a place that offer insights, tips and techniques from industry renowned fertility experts around the world.
- This is a place for people who don't want to feel like a victim to infertility and want to have a better quality of life by achieving your "other" life goals (non baby-making goals.)

This is my personal invitation for you to join my online support group!

Click here to join the online Facebook support group. And let me know that you got this information from my book.

**https://www.facebook.com/groups/NotYourTypicalFertilitySupportGroup/**

I look forward to interacting with you there!

# Foreword by Dr. Meera Shah

The journey to parenthood is rarely a straight path. Forecasting specific family planning timelines can often lead to disappointment—Mother Nature works in her own ways—mostly with no rhyme or reason. Most of us who live by the principle that hard work and effort result in reward feel a loss of control in the process of preparing to build a family. The burden of infertility has only increased over the past several decades—a result of delayed childbearing for a variety of socioeconomic reasons, changes in nutrition and environmental exposures, and other lifestyle changes. Simultaneously, society has shifted to more social isolation with advancements in technology and the introduction of social media—this, compounded with the stigma of infertility, has left couples feeling alone and lost in this journey. At least one in eight couples struggle with infertility—the psychological toll this takes on individuals and couples is profound. Until recently, there has been little attention focused on addressing the impact of infertility on rates of depression, anxiety, and marital conflict. This *needs* to change. And the journey of tackling infertility for couples *can* be different—it can be an opportunity to pause and reflect on what we have control over in our lives—as the serenity prayer teaches us, have the courage to change what we can and the serenity to accept what we cannot—it is an opportunity to support each other and perhaps bring us closer. The tools needed to have this outlook are what you will find in this book.

Crossing paths with Pradeepa was serendipitous, delightful, and awe-inspiring. As a newly practicing reproductive and infertility specialist, I found myself at a crossroads where I felt helpless in supporting my patients with the emotional rigor of the infertility journey. I could provide them the best treatments and medical advice, but that wasn't enough. They needed more—they needed a supporter, an advocate, and a motivational advisor—this is essentially what encompassed a "fertility coach". Unfamiliar with this term, Pradeepa taught me the difference between this and a traditional therapist. Pradeepa, with her unique experience through her own infertility journey, was perfectly suited for this role. She had experienced every possible setback one could face—pregnancy loss, countless failed IVF cycles including cycles using donor eggs, and ultimately she chose adoption to build her family. After experiencing the highs and lows of this journey and overcoming the countless obstacles, she realized that she was now equipped with something she had never had before—immense empathy, compassion, and the drive to help others struggling with infertility. It was unequivocally clear to me through many of our early conversations that she was genuinely passionate about this cause. She had found her true calling and now she was determined to spread her message and scale her vision to larger than what she ever imagined.

Since starting this path, Pradeepa has continued to make her impact both on small and large audiences. While continuing her individual coaching, she also hosted group workshops, developed her social media platforms, and recently delivered a TEDx talk in India, which was received with great enthusiasm. This book is her first published work, and the first of its kind to provide an interactive, practical guide to confront the many complex aspects of the infertility journey. It addresses both the female and male perspectives, as well as the couple together.

I look forward to sharing this book with my patients who are in various stages of their infertility treatment journey. I am so happy for anyone who comes across this gem!

Best of luck to all of you in this journey!

Sincerely,

Meera Shah, MD

Double board-certified Ob/Gyn and Reproductive Endocrinology and Infertility Specialist

Nova IVF, Mountain View, CA

# Foreword by Dr. Rinku Mehta

"It hurts the most when you have to start pretending it doesn't."

Infertility can be a lonely journey. Although one in eight couples suffers from infertility, most people don't talk about it. You get the invitation to the baby shower, but no one discusses if it was difficult to get there. Let's talk about it, let's eliminate the shame and stigma that comes with the burden of infertility.

I met Pradeepa when she came to visit me at my office to introduce herself. I was immediately struck by the kindness in her eyes and her desire to help people navigate the difficult path she has been through herself. It is difficult to share one's struggles with fertility, but telling one's story may help encourage other people. I, too, had suffered from infertility and even as a fertility specialist, I found myself walking in the shoes that my patients do and was an emotional mess through the process. For me it was a supportive relationship with my spouse and family that helped me through it, and I was fortunate to have been blessed with two children ultimately. I will however never forget those feelings of helplessness and devastation every time I got bad news.

Pradeepa's book, in my opinion, helps one recognize and acknowledge their feelings and open lines of communication with your spouse and loved ones. It is so easy to forget that your spouse is suffering through this too and may need as much support as you do. Additionally, it is so very important to have the same goals and be on the same page. Relationships suffer when the partners want different things and don't talk to each other. While having a child and building a family is a dream for most couples, if it doesn't happen, don't forget that you have each other. Being parents is a part of a relationship but should never define a relationship. Making time for each other and enjoying your togetherness makes the suffering of infertility a little more tolerable.

My advice to each patient that I see is to never forget about yourself and your spouse and continue to do things that you enjoy. Focus on your well-being first. It will give you the strength to deal with what comes your way.

Pradeepa's book is one such avenue to help couples navigate this journey, and it is my hope that many couples will take advantage of it.

Sincerely,

Rinku Mehta, MD

Reproductive Endocrinology and Infertility Specialist

Dallas IVF, Plano, TX`

# Introduction

Welcome to my first book! If your infertility SUCKS and you seem not in control, this is the right book for you.

I am so thrilled that you have decided to invest your time and energy to take care of your infertility struggles with this book! I will not promise that this book will help you get or stay pregnant. What I will promise is that this book will help you look at your infertility struggles through a different lens, get unstuck, move from being a victim to an owner, get clear on your path ahead, take care of your relationship struggles, and more importantly, live a GOOD life amid infertility.

This book will offer plenty of tips and techniques to help your infertility journey SUCK LESS!

## Who should read this book

- People who have just been diagnosed with infertility, those going through it and/or are about to or have had their first consult

- People who are getting ready to start a family and are experiencing some challenges of their own

- Friends and family members who are supporting loved ones on their infertility journey

- Generally curious minds who want to learn about and understand the emotional pain associated with infertility

I sincerely hope this book helps in your journey with infertility. My philosophy in anything I do in life, whether it's teaching, speaking, writing or coaching, is to make a positive impact on at least one person. I hope that person is you.

# Free 100 Questions eBook

## 100 Infertility Questions to Ask and Have Answered

An eBook by Pradeepa Narayanaswamy
Fertility Coach
Hello@PradeepaFertilityCoach.com
©www.PradeepaFertilityCoach.com

I would like to offer you the FREE digital version of *100 Infertility Questions to Ask and Have Answered*.

When it comes to dealing with infertility, first-time visits to fertility clinics can be thrilling and daunting at the same time. Many don't know what to expect and can often be unprepared for their first visit.

This list will arm you with questions you need to take to your doctor to prepare for a successful visit and also bring back great information that will help you make decisions about your next steps.

Even though the ultimate goal for the fertility clinic and the doctor visit is to get and stay pregnant with the prescribed treatments, the fertility journey and the treatment itself can be very complicated. These questions will help you make educated decisions to choose the option that best fits your needs and finances, as the treatments tend to be very expensive and often require out-of-pocket payment.

The book has a list of 100 questions that I have divided into different subsections. Each of these sections has a specific purpose that will help you ask pointed questions. These questions are not meant to be used verbatim, but rather are a helpful guideline when it comes to having a richer conversation with your fertility doctor and clinic.

Pick and choose the questions that are relevant for where you are in your journey and add anything from your own list before your visit.

https://pradeepafertilitycoach.com/free-e-book/

My best wishes for your fertility journey!

# Chapter 1

# Who Am I?

I'm a twelve-year infertility warrior turned fertility coach. My mission is to help YOUR infertility journey suck less, but apart from that, who is Pradeepa?

I'll share a little bit about me. I'm a fire dragon. That's actually my Chinese horoscope symbol and I really liked that because a dragon has both power and fire. This is not a destructive kind of fire, it's a fire that sparks people, and I use this to light the spark in my clients.

I love traveling around the world and I'm a vegetarian as well, so wherever I travel, I tend to find some local vegetarian dishes that I want to try.

Many of my friends and colleagues are appreciative of my listening skills—I am pretty good at listening, I'm not just a listener. I call myself a passionate listener. What a powerful phrase, *passionate listener*. This is a term coined by Harriet Lerner, a very famous psychologist, author, and speaker. According to her, passionate listening means listening with the same passion that we feel about wanting to be heard. That's who I am. It's not an innate skill. I worked really hard at it to become a passionate listener, to be a passionate listener for my clients, and it actually helps tremendously in coaching.

I am also a truth teller. I don't sugarcoat. I say what I see and what I sense and what I hear my clients as part of their service.

Last but not the least, there's one more detail I want to share about myself. Have you seen the TV show *Monk*? If you're not familiar with it, it's about a famous detective who solves amazing crimes. There's one characteristic that I learned after watching that show. Monk has OCD—Obsessive Compulsive Disorder. Everything needs to be perfectly organized for him. If he opens his clothes closet, his hangers need to be an equal distance from each other. Even if a hanger is only a quarter of an inch off, he has to move it. And that's how they show his OCD.

When I was reflecting on that characteristic, I got to thinking that I have a little bit of OCD as well. For example, I like my house very clean and organized. So after watching *Monk*, I did an experiment to test myself. I saw a few small food crumbs sitting on the floor and I waited to see how long I could ignore them. You know what? I was able to successfully ignore the crumbs for two minutes straight. After two minutes, I had to clean them up. After that, I started calling myself Ms. Monk.

So that's a little bit about me. I'm very excited that you have decided to give this book a try. I'm also very excited that I am going to be with you in your journey throughout this book.

# Chapter 2

# **Before We Begin**

Before we begin, I want to give you some pointers on how to best experience this book.

Find a quiet place to take the workbook assessment. This book is about your infertility journey and what you are going through and how you are feeling. It's about YOU. You don't want to be distracted.

There is a chapter for couples/partners. When you are reading that section, if you have a partner, try to read it together. That would be my strongest recommendation. Do it together as a couple.

Make sure you have a notebook and pen handy. There's going to be a lot of reflection. There are going to be a lot of things that you will want to note, so make sure you have a pen and paper handy.

Please make sure you have the course workbook printed out using the link at the end of this chapter. We are going to be using the workbook throughout the book. After every chapter, you will have an opportunity to do some activity in the workbook.

Next have a warm cup of your favorite drink. I also recommend that you have tissues with you because infertility can be hard depending upon where you are in your journey. Maybe you're just starting and don't know what this is going to be like for you. Maybe you are in the middle of your journey and going through all sorts of pains. Or you have exhausted all your possible options and are struggling to figure out what to do next. For these reasons and more, have some tissues handy.

1. Read the book in the suggested order. I have laid out the chapters in such a way that each one builds upon previous chapters.
2. After every lesson there'll be a workbook activity, and I will walk you through what needs to be done in the workbook. It's best to do it then and there if possible.
3. Again, if you haven't printed out your workbook, make sure you do because that's where you're going to get the most out of the book.
4. Pause and take as much time as needed between the chapters. Infertility is not an easy thing. It can be a very tough, painful journey for many of you. This book will lead you through a lot of reflection, which may bring out a lot of emotions. Honor those and reflect as much as you can, pausing as much as you need to.
5. Continue reflecting as much as possible.

Here is a brief overview of the various chapters in this book.

1. Why do I care about infertility? I'll be sharing my story and talking about why I care about supporting people going through infertility.

2. What is infertility? I'm going to talk a little bit about what infertility is, and I'll share some quick facts with you. When I discovered these things for the first time, I thought, *Wow, this is big*, so I wanted to share them with you.

3. As a woman, what is it like to be on this journey? How are you showing up on this journey? What can you do?

4. As a man, what is it like to be on this journey? How are you showing up on this journey? What can you do?

5. As a couple, how does infertility affect couples and their relationship? I'll share tips and techniques to help restore the relationship.

6. Family and friends—how can we forget our friends and family? These are the people who really care about us and love us. They are struggling to see how they can support you, and this chapter is perfect for them. What are the things to do and say, and what are some of the things not to do or say?

7. Bringing it all together.

8. Next steps and some useful resources. We will cover some important next steps for you, and I will leave you with some wonderful resources that are going to help educate you about infertility.

So these are the different chapters in this book. Now that you're coming to the end of this chapter, I'm just going to repeat it one more time. Don't hate me, please. Make sure to download the workbook using the link below.

Once downloaded, please print it out.

**https://pradeepafertilitycoach.com/infertility-can-suck-less-workbook/**

# Chapter 3

# **Why Do I Care About Infertility?**

Why do I care about infertility?

My personal experience with infertility opened my eyes to the extreme need for support and service in a world where many people are also experiencing infertility and going through their own journeys. I understand that this is a process people don't want to talk about or don't know who to talk to.

But I want to talk to you about that and share my story. To do that, I want to take you back to the year 2000.

That's when I got married.

Originally from India, in September of 2000, I arrived in New York—Long Island, to be exact—and life was good. Lots of fun, lots of joy.

Several years passed.

If you are from an Indian family, or even a Southeast Asian family, after a few years people start asking these questions: When are you going to have a child? What's the delay?

I finally got pregnant in 2006.

We were very happy.

It took a while, but finally we did it. We shared our pregnancy news with some close friends and family.

Little did I know at the time that this pregnancy was going to change my life forever. In fact, it changed after only eleven weeks. During the middle of the night I experienced an ache in my stomach, and I immediately knew something wasn't right.

I had a miscarriage.

That was the first really hard thing I had to go through in my life.

I was in so much grief, so much pain.

I still can remember those days after the miscarriage. Every morning I would get calls from my parents and my mother-in-law from India. I hated those calls, to be honest.

They reminded me so much of the loss I had suffered. I just wanted to disappear from the face of the Earth and run away from all the pain. I was in grief, and it took a while for me to come out of that. But I did come out of it, and I got pregnant again for a second time, only to lose the baby again. And it happened a third time.

I miscarried again. That's when I talked to the doctor. The doctor said he didn't know what was going on and referred me to a specialist. At that time, I lived in Minneapolis, and I was referred to Dr. Bruce Campbell. For the first time in my life, I heard the words *assisted reproduction*, and I became curious. I thought, *Wow, there is assistance available for reproduction*.

I started to feel hopeful that maybe this doctor could help me, even though we didn't know what was going on. After all, this was something I couldn't do without assistance. I needed assistance for reproducing. *Sigh!*

I'm a person who doesn't give up easily. We met with Dr. Campbell, and he was such a wonderful person. I still remember him. He gave us all the protocols. Some of the initial treatments didn't work, so we were put on more rigorous treatments. The first one they started me on was IUI—intrauterine insemination. You might be familiar with this if you are going through fertility treatments. We had three cycles, and they were back to back-to-back failures.

Then we got together again with Dr. Campbell, and he suggested that we try IVF—in vitro fertilization. Even today, IVF is the gold standard for fertility treatments.

I'm the type of person who reads articles and does research. After checking into IVF, I got excited because the information and facts I read about it were more positive. The success rates compared to those for IUI were significant.

Let me tell you a little bit about it. It's not just a one-time process where you go to the doctor's office and get the treatment done. It's rigorous and a very long process. Each cycle is a few months long, with lots of injections, lots of medications, lots of treatments, lots of blood work and absolute discipline. It's expected. You know what, those were all fine with me. Those were all procedural things, and I am a pretty strong person. I knew I could do it, I could handle it—and I did. I just went with it.

I handled every bit of these treatments with so much optimism, so much hope. I was determined to get through the journey.

I completed the IVF cycle, and finally my day arrived! The morning came when I would get my blood work done, and in the afternoon the doctor would call me and tell me that I was pregnant. I still remember that day. I couldn't sleep the previous night because I was super excited. I got up early in the morning because I typically went for treatments before going to work. I was up at five, got dressed, got ready, and was the first person at the clinic when they opened, ready for them to take my blood. I was that eager. I was that committed. I got my blood test done and then went to work.

I was pretty distracted that day. I had a Blackberry phone back then, and I was looking at it every two minutes. Was my doctor calling? I knew he wouldn't typically call in the morning just like the nurse said, but what if...what if he got the results sooner and he just wanted to share the good news with me? *You're pregnant—congratulations! It worked!*

It was so distracting looking at my phone the whole day. However, late in the afternoon, for whatever reason, I missed the phone call. I recognized the phone number immediately because I knew the clinic's number by heart, since I had called it so many times. With my hands trembling I called my voicemail and listened to Dr. Campbell's message. And all I heard was, "Pradeepa, I am very sorry..." As I heard that, I saw my phone falling from my hand. Literally, it fell.

Tears started flowing uncontrollably.

I couldn't stop it. It was unstoppable.

I thought this was my day. It was not. Then I realized I was at work. I picked up my phone and wiped my tears away fast. I ran to the desk, grabbed my bag, and ran outside.

My colleague was sitting at the next desk and looked at me like, *what's going on*? I just ran as fast as I could to my car. I didn't want to be there. My first IVF failure, even after I gave myself over completely to that process. I grieved for a while. The so-called gold standard DID NOT work for me. What would I do? I felt lost.

But like I said, I don't give up easily. I went back to Dr. Campbell's office and asked him what we should we do. He suggested that we change the protocol. We tried again.

It didn't work. We tried again and again. First, second, third, fourth, fifth, sixth, seventh, eighth tries. Eight back-to-back IVF failures. It was EXHAUSTING!

It was as if every time I started this treatment, I was climbing the stairs of a building thirty stories high, only to fall down face-first from the window and break into pieces. I had to pick myself up and climb those stairs all over again. And that was my life with all my IVF treatments and failures.

I just gave up.

All the medications and injections affected me physically, as did the hormones, all the losses, and all the failures. It affected me emotionally and mentally, and it affected me spiritually quite a bit too. I avoided going to India for four years, giving all sorts of BS reasons why I couldn't go. You know why I didn't want to go? Because I didn't want my husband to face the inevitable questions.

At work, I was faking it and wearing a mask like everything was perfect. Nobody knew anything about my personal struggles with infertility or that my relationship with my husband was struggling.

I felt like I was on an island struggling alone and feeling lonely. I didn't have anybody who could relate to what I was going through.

I didn't know what to ask of my husband. He didn't know how to support me, and we were not communicating with each other.

Our intimacy and our relationship were struggling.

I was so lonely.

It was so hard. I was in so much pain.

I was desperate. I was jealous. People all around me were getting pregnant. All my friends and family members who had gotten married after me were all getting pregnant, having babies and birthday parties.

I wondered, *Why not me? Why did you choose for me to be this way?*

That was my life for eight years with various treatments. You know what the most frustrating part about my infertility journey was? Our diagnosis was labeled UNEXPLAINED INFERTILITY! It means, "There is no apparent reason for your infertility." It was difficult, maddening, and frustrating. I'd gone through all the possible tests and procedures there were; the only thing doctors hadn't done was cut open my body. My life completely changed. It was SO hard to live with that diagnosis.

After the eighth failure with four different doctors, my husband suggested that we try once more. I had never said this, but I told my husband, no, I couldn't do it anymore. He respected my decision. That's when we mutually decided to go the adoption route, and we started the paperwork immediately.

It took me more than three years to truly move on and make peace with my infertility.

I struggled through a lot, and I learned a lot from my journey about what to do and what not to do.

I know how sucky this journey is. It truly sucked for me.

I wish I had a Pradeepa back then supporting me. I am sure my journey would have been different, and my attitude would have been different. I would not have made those same mistakes and would have had a more positive experience.

Call me crazy, but I am grateful for my infertility because it gave me a bigger purpose in life: to support others going through infertility. That's why I became a fertility coach. I coach both individuals and couples who want to take control of their lives and stay energized and positive as they move forward with infertility.

I am doing what I'm doing today—becoming a fertility coach—to help men and women and couples so their journey doesn't have to suck that much. You know what my mission is?

**My mission is to help YOUR infertility journey suck less.**

I cannot say it will be "suck free" because there will be some level of your journey that's going to suck.

There is a silver lining to my story. We adopted our son Kartik.

He just turned seven. He came into our lives three years ago. I'm a mother, and he truly changed me for the better.

Like I said, my journey sucked, and when I was going through it, I was just going and going and going, but yet I was completely STUCK. Not stopping for a minute and not thinking or reflecting. Never. I never did that. I never dreamt about my ideal journey. I never dreamt it. But you know what? No matter where you are in your journey today, whether you are just starting, whether you are in the middle of your treatments, or you are an IVF veteran like me, I've been where you are in this journey. I want you to take a moment and dream your ideal journey. This will help you be more intentional about your journey.

# I invite you to dream your IDEAL JOURNEY!!!

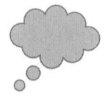

- You can write.
- You can draw or paint.
- You can sing.
- You can dance.
- You can write a song.
- Anything that helps your creative channel to DREAM!!

To do that, go to the link below to download your copy of the workbook. Once downloaded, please print it out.

**https://pradeepafertilitycoach.com/infertility-can-suck-less-workbook/**

# Chapter 4

# **What Is Infertility?**

I hope you had an amazing dream of your ideal fertility journey. We are now into the next chapter, which is an introduction to infertility. This is where I'm going to share some things with you, even though I'm not a medical doctor.

I'm just going to give you a little bit of information from the medical side of the house. It's important to understand what infertility is. I'll explain it in my own terms. If you are having regular sexual intercourse for twelve months and trying for a child but it's just not happening, you may have infertility. Also, growing up, if your body or your partner's body was physically impaired and this is not allowing you to have a child, that is also termed as infertility.

I'm going to share some quick facts about infertility. Do you know how many couples go through infertility?

One in eight couples go through infertility, and that's a lot. If you're in a room with ten couples who are in the age range of having a child, there is a high chance that one of them is going through infertility. The majority of the time, infertility and the challenges associated with it are focused mainly on women. But it's not just the female factor: 33 percent is attributed to the female factor, 33 percent is

17

attributed to the, male factor and the remaining 33 percent is a combination or it's unexplained, just like our diagnosis.

Did you know that 11.9 percent (almost 12 percent) of women actually go through infertility treatments in their life? That's twelve women out of every hundred, and that's a lot.

Let's take couples between twenty-nine and thirty-three years of age with normal functioning reproductive systems who don't have any challenges or any previous issues. Did you know that their chance of conceiving in any given month is only between 20 and 25 percent? I didn't know that, and that's a very small percentage.

After trying for six months, only 60 percent of them get pregnant without any medical assistance. That means 40 percent of our population goes through some kind of medical assistance to get pregnant.

Why am I talking about all these statistics? When I was going through this, I didn't know these facts. Many of us think it's just us going through this dreadful time, especially if it's a really hard journey. I'm not trying to minimize your situation and your journey, but this list of facts actually gives you some perspective. You're not by yourself. You're not alone.

There are so many people in the world going through infertility, and these are just some data points for you. **This is a complex, massive problem**. One of my male friends who went through fertility challenges himself told me these exact words. This is a complex, massive problem that we just don't realize exists.

You know how the world deals with the topic of infertility? We don't talk about it. It's a hush-hush, taboo subject in many cultures, including where I come from in India; it's a very sensitive subject. There is so much stigma around it. Let me be very honest with all of you. Until my OB-GYN told me that I should go see a fertility specialist, I was naive and didn't even know that fertility challenges and treatments existed. While growing up, I never heard anybody in my family or outside my family talking about it openly. People don't like to talk about this. And many people don't know how to talk about it. There is no screening for infertility. There is a big lack of awareness.

And that is the next challenge!

If you don't have the awareness about it or want to talk about it, how do your support someone going through fertility challenges? What do you say to them and what do you not to say to them? I have a chapter dedicated to friends and family with plenty of tips and techniques to support your loved ones going through infertility.

It's time for the workbook. Go to the link below to download your copy of the workbook. Once downloaded, please print it out. In the workbook, capture where you are in your fertility journey as well as any additional questions or facts you want to find answers to.

**https://pradeepafertilitycoach.com/infertility-can-suck-less-workbook/**

# Chapter 5

# As a Woman Going Through Infertility

As a woman, I went through a very long, hard, and painful fertility journey. It may not be the same for you, but I am sure my experiences will resonate with you. There are many given factors with infertility, and I'll share from my experience some of the givens in my journey.

There were so many unknowns—I really didn't know what was going to happen, what treatment would work for me, or what else I needed to do to make this successful. And that was so frustrating. Really, really frustrating! My path ahead was unclear. It was as if I was wearing Vaseline-smeared glasses—no matter how hard I tried to clean the glasses, it just wouldn't go away. I felt so stuck and so desperate to know what I should do next. That really, really sucked my energy. My energy was very low.

It was hard knowing that I didn't have any control of my fertility journey. I was just going and going and going, and even though the process was constantly ongoing, I was stuck because things were not moving ahead, even though the months were moving and the years were passing. There were so many failures in my journey, and I was stuck with infertility. It was as if I was stuck in quicksand that just sucked me farther and farther down. I was desperate to find a twig to hold onto, to climb up. And there was so much guilt; even though they couldn't find any real problem in me, still my mind kept asking, *why not*? Why is this happening to me? What is wrong with me? It was as if I had this big question mark on my head all the time.

For many of us, situational depression happens. It's not clinical depression, it's situational specifically because of infertility. That's the situation.

And if you are going through fertility treatments, you know injections are a BIG given—there's no way it'll work without them. There are so many injections; it's not just one injection and you're done, it's multiple injections in a day, and you have to be absolutely disciplined about it. Absolutely disciplined. And for me, it was eight years of that discipline with treatments.

In the previous chapter I talked a little bit about my journey, but in this chapter, as a woman I want to take you through the different emotions I experienced during my journey. To do that, I'm going to use a tool called a journey map; since my treatment journey was eight years long, I cannot show all of it on this page. I'm just picking out one small segment of it. It's my first donor cycle, so this is actually my sixth IVF attempt, and here is the map.

Once I did this map, it helped me reflect on my own gaps and actions. It helped me realize where I was stuck and revealed my motivations and the decisions I was making. The benefit of doing this journey map will help one take control of their own actions and change as desired.

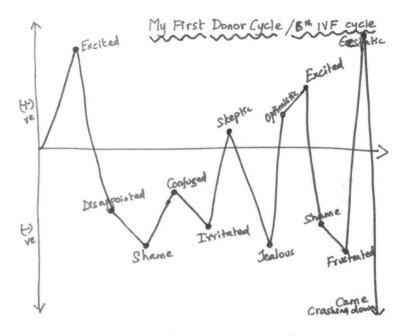

On the bottom are all the positive emotions. You'll also see all my negative emotions for the cycle. We saw a new doctor, Dr. Sherbahn, who had a very good track record. I did all my research and I was very, very excited for my journey. I was excited to meet him for the first time, just to hear what he could offer that was different that could help me finally get pregnant. So, I'm just going to express my emotions—I'm very excited here. That's what this is all about.

When he was going through our records in our first meeting, he noticed that I had gone through so many IVF treatments that failed. He immediately recommended donor eggs.

BOOM!

I was so disappointed after hearing that. This is it. My eggs are faulty. It doesn't work anymore. I was SO ashamed. I was also very confused and started coming up with these "what if" stories in my head. What if I use donor eggs and end up conceiving, then go through the whole pregnancy term and have a baby—the baby's not going to look like me. That baby is not going to have any of my traits or characteristics. That was my fear. I was so confused. And knowing that my husband's sperm was still going to be used, I got mad at him for that. I was really mad, irritated, and annoyed. Here I am going through all these things in the IVF cycle, and now I have to use donor eggs. That in itself was a big blow for me. And nothing would change for him. Nothing would be different for him. I WAS SO MAD! I didn't talk to him for a few days after that, and I was constantly getting irritated during every interaction with him.

I had to get over the idea of using donor eggs because I was becoming a person that no one would want to be around. Somehow, I had to make up my mind about this. As I said previously, I don't give up easily, but still it took a while and I had to do it on my own.

As we were starting my donor IVF cycle, life happened. Guess what? One of my close friends announced her pregnancy.

I was happy, but I was also sad, angry, and jealous. I couldn't help it. It was really hard knowing that I was jealous of my friend's pregnancy. There was nothing malicious behind my feelings, yet I was still beating myself up for having those emotions. What kind of a friend am I? I am not a good friend, I am a MONSTER! And that made it even harder to know what to do next.

Somehow, I had to get ready for my donor cycle and try really hard to be positive. I saw myself having fun going over the donor profiles. My husband asked me to make the decision as to which profile I wanted. He did not take any part in looking over or selecting the donor. I went through the donor profiles to select somebody who I felt would be a good match for me. And you know what, I got more excited because the procedures were in progress.

The only thing I had left to do was to go for the implantation of the embryos, which I did, and then I went for my blood work. In the meantime, of course, life didn't stop for me at work. I again had a fake mask on, pretending life was great for me. I felt a lot of shame. Again, in an attempt to avoid that feeling, I pretended that everything was fine with me. Nobody knew what was going on. Even after all those tries and all those cycles and all the things that were going on with me, I was still so ashamed about my infertility. I was holding onto it, which really distracted me at work. My colleagues had kids, and they talked about their kids, which sometimes felt frustrating to me.

But this time, after going for my blood work, I was positive I was pregnant. In fact, this was the only time in my IVF journey when I actually got a positive pregnancy result—

and I was pregnant with twins. I was *super* excited. I was so thrilled, and I thought, *Wow, this is it.* All the disappointment, the shame, the confusion, the meditation, the skepticism slowly started to disappear and drift away and was replaced by my excitement.

This time we were very careful. We didn't tell anybody our news. We just wanted to make sure everything would be okay, and this is where the universe tested me again. A few weeks after that positive test result, I knew that something was not right in my body. I immediately went to the doctor again. After some tests, he announced that I was slowly losing the babies. They were not going to survive. The doctor wasn't hearing their heartbeats anymore. My entire world came crashing down completely.

If this is where I wanted to stop talking about this journey, you'd see most of it as an emotional roller coaster. And I'm just talking about a very small cycle among all the different treatments that I had.

To put a little bit of color into this chart, I found emotion stickers at Michaels. You can find these emotion stickers at many different arts and crafts stores. So when I was excited, I represented it with one of the stickers on the chart.

After that, I was disappointed and ashamed because it was suggested that I use donor eggs instead of my own. Because of this, I was frowning and very confused—that's where the frowny sticker would go. With the feeling of shame, I was totally irritated and annoyed with my husband as well as confused. I was slowly becoming a little bit skeptical, and then when my friend announced her pregnancy, I became jealous.

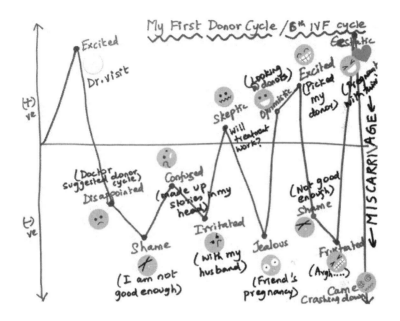

That's how this map shows my wide range of emotions. And then the smile emotion returns when I became more optimistic as I started looking at the donor profiles. At that point, I started smiling a little bit again, and then when I picked the person whose eggs we would use, I got really excited, and I was all smiles. Then the big shame factor came in again because at work I really couldn't share how I felt. It was so frustrating for me to have to hear people's baby stories and see pregnant women at work. That was really hard on me.

Then I got pregnant with twins, and I was all smiles. I wanted to put another smiley sticker on because that's how happy I was. But then that was taken away from me when I lost the twins. You can use many types of stickers to show your emotions, and I wanted to show you mine as an example.

This is my journey map just on my first donor cycle. The reason I'm using these stickers is that they help to capture my emotions at the time and show how up and down my journey was, and it can help you as well. Understanding the various emotions at different points can help you truly acknowledge what you are going through. It can also help you be more intentional about how you want to deal with that emotion and what you want to do next.

You can see I spent a long time maintaining that discipline. There were so many ancillary things too, like acupuncture, yoga, diet, tea, and many more that are advertised targeting women. And I've tried all of them in desperation. I mentioned that my journey had many emotional roller coaster rides, and even though my journey map only shows a very short period of time, you can still see the many ups and downs I experienced.

On my SUCK-O-METER, my suckiness level was at an all-time high. It was through the roof.

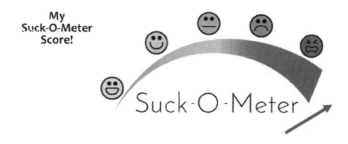

**My
Suck-O-Meter
Score!**

It was so high that I think the meter would break if I had an actual physical meter. That's how it was for me. I was lonely, and I was ashamed. I was fearful because time was running out for me. I was so worried. I was so desperate. I kept thinking, *please let this be my time*, and when things didn't happen, I was so frustrated. I felt inadequate, guilty, and jealousy. There were just so many emotions. It was definitely a roller coaster ride for me, and it was an eventful ride.

I would love for you to take a moment to draw a journey map on a recent event with your fertility journey and see how you can map your various emotions. This exercise will help you reflect on your own gaps and actions. It can help you understand where you are stuck and how your motivations and decisions are contributing to that. The benefit of doing this journey map is that it will help you take control of your actions and identify changes that you would like to make moving forward.

This is a very popular tool that I use with many of my clients, and they often tell me how revealing it is. They learn so much about themselves.

You can use this chart below for your list of various emotions.

| Desperate | Sad | Anger | Frustrated | Lonely | Irritated |
|---|---|---|---|---|---|
| Jealous | Inadequate | Shameful | Confused | Annoyed | Optimistic |
| Curious | Fearful | Hopeful but Guarded | Guilty | Grief | Worried |
| Disappointed | Happy | Excited | Nervous | Terrified | Tensed |
| Heartbroken | Depressed | Mad | Rage | Scared | Joy |

Go to this link to download your copy of the workbook to do the journey map. Once downloaded, please print it out.

**https://pradeepafertilitycoach.com/infertility-can-suck-less-workbook/**

I hope you are able to draw your own journey map and capture some emotions. What was an *aha moment* for you? What did you learn from drawing your journey map?

Take a moment and think about these questions.

I wanted to discuss another aspect of my journey—what did I do to cope with the emotional aspect? How did I cope with my journey at the time? Can you guess what I did? Netflix.

That was my coping mechanism.

I came home and binge-watched Netflix even before binge-watching was coined as a term. I used to think that if Netflix was observing my viewing pattern, they would have called it "Pradeepa-watching" and then changed the term to "binge-watching" later. I was just trying to forget everything that was happening in my life all day, every day. I was a couch potato, which was not healthy, but that's how I chose to cope with it. That's how I chose to be numb. That's how I chose to ignore it. I had this big thing going on in my life with all these emotions and this roller coaster journey, and none of that was healthy. There are many things I should have said no to, but I didn't.

Being on Google all day and every day made me a Google expert, desperately searching for answers. Is drinking this tea, taking this supplement, eating this type of food helpful or harmful? I even found a suggestion to eat fries from a specific McDonald's restaurant. It was madness. There was so much conflicting information, and I had no idea which I should listen to.

I joined a bunch of support groups, especially online groups. Those groups only brought me down. It didn't help to compare my test results and numbers with other people's. I'd just tell them my HCG number and ask, "What do you think? Do I have a chance?" Things like that. I was desperate!

I used to do that all the time, and it didn't really help. All those people in the groups were not doctors, they're all other people just like me going through infertility, and I was desperately looking for answers in the wrong places. Some support groups gave me medical advice, like, *have you tried this procedure? Ask your doctor to do this because it worked for me*. These groups are not run by medical doctors and it's a bad idea to take those suggestions. Again, I was desperate to find THE silver bullet that would finally work for me.

I was trying to find solace in other people's failures. It sounds mean, because of what I was going through at the time, that was my reality, and now I'm admitting it. Hanging out with family, friends, and colleagues who just brought me down or reminded me of what I didn't have and desperately desired didn't really help me. I wish I had said no to them, but I didn't. These things would be on my "no" list.

So here are some things I certainly wish I had said yes to. Self-care—I never cared about myself at that time. I never loved me. I was angry at myself all the time. I hated me. Self-love is important. Intentional acceptance of the situation and reality. For example, just practice by saying something like this: "This journey sucks my energy and I know it." Even just saying that out loud, you're actually accepting it—accepting the reality. If you are an extravert who likes to hang out with people, go hang out with people you absolutely love and who love you back, as well as those who do not remind you of your fertility struggles. In general, just hang out with more positive and uplifting people. If you're an introvert, maybe take a nap or read a favorite book. Learn a new craft, something that you always wanted to learn. For example, ethnic cooking, painting, photography, coloring, poetry, anything that you've wanted to do. Say yes to that. Say yes to recording your suckiness score and the suck-o-meter. See where you are. And see how you can bring that score down even a teensy bit.

Do some charity work, volunteer for a nonprofit, catch up on chores or find activities that you truly enjoy. For me, like I said earlier, I'm Ms. Monk, so I like to clean and organize my home, and that is something that relaxes me. Join a support group that truly supports you, uplifts you, and cheers you up, not one that brings you down. Talk to a professional fertility coach like me, someone who has experienced infertility and can offer you a safe space to explore your feelings. I am sure as a woman you are doing this already because I was—talk to a medical professional about getting tips to improve your fertility. Is there anything you can do? These are the tips I wish I had when I was going through this journey. I will see you in the workbook part.

If you don't have the workbook, go to the link below to download your copy. Once downloaded, please print it out.

**https://pradeepafertilitycoach.com/infertility-can-suck-less-workbook/**

# Chapter 6

# **Are Men the Forgotten Entity?**

Welcome to the "As a Man" chapter. Let me share two quick facts with you. Did you know the fertility industry is expected to be valued at more than $21 billion globally by 2020? This whopping number was in an article published in *Newsweek* magazine. And the second fact is that the male partner is either the sole or a contributing cause in about 40 percent of infertility cases. This is a fact from the American Society of Reproductive Medicine (ASRM).

There is a reason why I put the above two facts together. The majority of the time, the $21 billion industry that I'm talking about focuses almost exclusively on women. That's a lot. And what about men? You are also a contributing factor, as shown by ASRM's report. Men are often a forgotten or an ignored entity when it comes to infertility. Initially when I started working with people going through fertility challenges, I was primarily focusing on women. But very quickly my perspective changed because ever since I started talking to their male partners, I started seeing that they were struggling too. However, too often we don't include them. We don't even ask how they are feeling.

They're forgotten. They go through this just like women do. They may show it differently. They may not be as emotional as we women are, but they go through the pain

35

as well; they go through the loss. They go through the emotions.

I'll talk about some of the given factors for men. The majority of the time, if they are NOT dealing with male infertility factors, they take on a supportive role. There are two aspects to this supportive role:

1. They must support their partner because the partner is going through all sorts of treatments and injections and hormonal changes, as well as moods and reactions to medications—everything.
2. They are feeling any suckiness that's happening in their journey, too.

They need to take on those two roles, which they have to execute beautifully. Actually, that's the big challenge for them. And men are oftentimes in the ancillary role. They are the ones who are giving injections. My husband used to be so prompt and disciplined. He would always make sure he came home from work in time for my treatment—if my injection needed to be given at 7 p.m., he'd be home by 6:30 p.m. And if you're a male partner or if you're a woman reading this, I'm sure you can understand what I'm talking about.

Men may not be going through the treatments themselves, but many of the men that I talk to *care*. They care about their partners and they get frustrated. They really want to take the pain off their wife. They cannot do anything to fix the situation right now, and they feel like everything is on their head. Men want to share in this but they can't, that's the reality of the situation.

It impacts their sex life and their social life. One of my male friends who experienced infertility with his partner calls infertility a complex massive problem. We don't talk about this subject, but do you know what? It's a complex massive problem and there are many emotions that men experience going through infertility. They have anger toward the process because there is only so much they can control. Men tend to be fixers in general, but this is something they cannot fix, which results in anger. There is also frustration—*"Oh my God, I have no idea what my wife is going through or what my female partner is going through"*, which creates frustration.

One of my clients wrote to me the other day that they just failed their eighth IUI. He was so worried about his wife. He was feeling so helpless and had no idea how to support her.

One of my other male clients would go to the shooting range and shoot his gun to blow off steam (not recommended). There are a lot of different ways that men tend to express some of their emotions. There are a lot more emotions that we typically don't talk about. How about fear? How about shame? Shame comes up, especially when the male factor is involved. There's male pride, right? That male pride is destroyed now because he has a problem with his fertility, his reproductive viability.

Besides anger and frustration, there's the feeling of guilt. *"Oh my God, I cannot support my wife here"* or *"I have a problem. I don't know how to go about this. And I feel guilty."* And of course, there's grief and worry—all those emotions are there for men too.

I want to share five tips, five things to do that will help you take control of your journey. Even though you are in this with your partner, sometimes you have to take care of yourself.

**Number one**, be intentional. Be intentional about your role in this journey. One of my friends who went through this called himself the chief relaxation officer. I love that nickname he gave himself. By the way, he's the CEO of a company. So, he thinks from that perspective and talks in those terms. Maybe you want to call yourself a chief movie planning officer, maybe you're a chief romantic data officer. Whatever is right for you.

**Number two,** be more intentional about your role in that journey and please, *please* don't forget to get support from your friends or your family members or even from support groups. Oftentimes, men tend to sweep the idea of support under the rug, like, *"Eh, I don't have to. No, it's all right. Everything is okay."* But when you're going through something like this, everything is not okay. Don't sweep your feelings under the rug. And I use this analogy: If you keep sweeping your dirt under the rug, you know what's going to happen? Eventually when you lift the rug, it's going to be a stinky bomb. It's going to be a stinky bomb and that stink is not good for yourself or your relationship. So, don't sweep your emotions under the rug. Get support and do things together.

**Number three**, this is a tip that one of my clients gave me. He does things with his very close friends, and there's one gentleman in particular who he'll do things with, like going for a golf outing or going to see a movie or whatever. They don't set time to talk about the struggles; instead, they have a casual conversation. "Hey man, our last IVF didn't work out. You know, it's really sucking. I have no idea how to support my wife." It doesn't have to be a serious sit-down conversation. Sometimes men don't care about those things. They're not comfortable with those things. So go out and do something, and then also talk about it.

**Number four**, talk to a fertility coach like myself, who has truly experienced this and understands what you are going through because I have been on the other side as well. I have gone through infertility, and I can offer you a safe space to explore your feelings and determine how you need to move forward.

**Number five**, talk to a doctor. Talk to your doctor and see whether he/she can offer you any tips to improve your fertility. You don't have to tell anyone. Women proactively go and talk to their doctors to ask about infertility; they also join different support groups and ask things like does this herb work? Does this tea work? We are really good at that. But men typically don't do that. For those men, I would recommend you talk to your doctor.

## Things to do

| 01 | 02 | 03 | 04 | 05 |
|---|---|---|---|---|
| Be intentional about your role in this journey | Get support from your close friends/family or support groups | Do things with your friends & still be able to talk about your struggles | Talk to a professional fertility coach who can offer a safe space to explore feelings & help move forward | Talk to a medical professional about getting tips to improve your fertility |
| Examples: Chief Relaxation Officer, Chief Movie Planning Officer | | | | |

I talked about things to do. Now I'm going to share five things not to do. Please don't get drunk or do drugs or smoke, they're not good for you. And don't do something stupid like releasing your aggression at a shooting range or race car driving or going skydiving or anything like that. It may not be the right time to do those things. Also, avoid extreme stress and constant intense feelings. Talk to somebody about how you feel.

This is something that I heard from one of my friends: don't try to prove your manliness with other women. It not only hurts you, it hurts your relationship immensely. And last but not least, don't wear tight underwear. That's why a lot of men who are going through fertility challenges switch to wearing briefs, including my husband.

# Things to Avoid

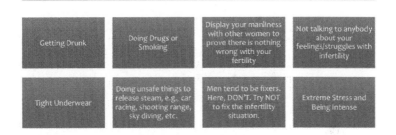

I'll talk to you further in the workbook section.

If you don't have the workbook yet, go to the link below to download your copy of the workbook. Once downloaded, please print it out.

[https://pradeepafertilitycoach.com/infertility-can-suck-less-workbook/](https://pradeepafertilitycoach.com/infertility-can-suck-less-workbook/)

# Chapter 7

## The Invisible Wall Between Couples

We are now in the "As a Couple" chapter. Like I mentioned before, it's best to work through this chapter as a couple.

I want to share a few stories here. Does this situation sound familiar? Maybe you miscarried or you lost a baby. You're crying and so emotional, and you just want to be left alone. You're grieving so much, and your husband may be silent because he just doesn't know how to support you.

Have you been in this situation as a wife? You go through a treatment or procedure by yourself. For some reason your husband couldn't come with you, and your doctor tells you so many things that it was information overload.

You then come home and tell your husband all this information. *This is what my doctor told me. This is what we need to do. This is what we have to take. This is where we have to go. This is the medicine I need to order, this is the injection that I must take. This is the next step, this is the next time I must go for an appointment.*

For the husband, it's like, "Whoa, that's a lot of information", and your husband may seem to check out. If you're a man, do you check out when you receive an information overload? As a couple during infertility challenges, do you find fault in each other no matter what? Even for smaller things here and there.

It's not uncommon. It is common with infertility. Making a baby isn't sexy, it's stressful. It's really hard. And of course, it's miserable and robotic, knowing there are specific times you have to do it. You're losing intimacy here and it's not for pleasure anymore. And there is the constant stress of the treatments and the repeated disappointments that can totally strain your relationship.

Women may feel more irritable and emotional, like a volcano that's about to burst, and her partner may feel helpless and worried. Women's emotions can go up and down—positive one minute and negative the next, fluctuating up and down. You never know what's going to show up. It can be tough on the partner, and most importantly when you're going through something as difficult as this, couples don't have proper tools to support and communicate with each other. Maybe they're not taught these things while growing up. Do you know what the outcome of this can be? It happened to me. There is an invisible wall that's growing tall and strong and thick between the couple and it affects the intimacy and relationship a lot.

I want to talk about four toxins that can develop in a relationship.

A study was done by Drs. John and Julie Gottman of The Gottman Institute, in which they talk about four toxins that appear in any relationship:

1. Criticism
2. Defensiveness
3. Contempt
4. Stonewalling

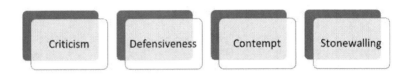

Criticism:

Let's talk about criticism a little bit and think about your situation with infertility. When this happens, criticism is basically attacking the person rather than the situation: "What's wrong with you? Why are you being so stupid? You never think of me, you're so selfish. I'm going through all this." You're attacking the person rather than the situation. This is criticism, and this is one of the four toxins.

Defensiveness:

Number two is defensiveness. Defensiveness is a typical response to criticism. Here, what people are doing is fishing for excuses to play the innocent victim. When people start making excuses, it tells the other person that we are not taking their concerns seriously. Or worse, we are not taking responsibility for our mistakes. Defensiveness is almost always an unsuccessful strategy and only escalates conflict. When you're being defensive, it's another way of blaming your partner.

Contempt:

Number three is contempt. It's the worst, and Drs. John and Julie Gottman call it the most poisonous of all four toxins. Contempt in your relationship, sarcasm, belittling, name-calling, cynicism, hostile humor—all these are part of contempt. It actually conveys disgust and condescension, and when there is contempt in a relationship, it is harmful for physical well-being as well. It's that harmful. When you keep belittling somebody, when you're speaking sarcastically, when you are name-calling, when you are being a cynic, it affects the other person's health a lot, and there is a study that proves it.

There are negative thoughts constantly going on. That actually triggers contempt, and do you know why we have continual negative thoughts about somebody? Because we are not communicating, we have unresolved differences in our relationship and we are not talking about them on a regular basis.

**Contempt is the single greatest predictor of divorce today.** If you see a couple going to a divorce lawyer or ending up in divorce, 90 percent of the time there was contempt in their relationship. This is research that I personally did by talking to different people across the United States.

The question I asked was, "How is infertility affecting your relationship?" These were some of the answers I collected, and contempt seemed to play a big role in these relationships.

Names of the people quoted below are not included to respect their privacy.

"Of course, infertility was not our only problem, but I do think it played a large part in ending the relationship."

"This process truly is a make or break on relationships. It broke mine."

"My husband got a job in North Carolina and I still lived in New York. As much as I didn't like being apart, I think it helped."

"I literally just had a fight with my partner. Every time I bring it up, he doesn't want to talk about it."

"The emotional and financial strain is really pushing us to our limit."

"It's awful! IVF is so hard financially, emotionally, and physically, and a lot of men don't understand that."

"Making a baby isn't sexy. It isn't fun. Especially when you've got infertility. It's stressful. It's hard. It's hormonal. It's just miserable. I don't have proper support."

"The constant stress of it all has definitely strained our relationship. I think when you struggle with fertility it can tend to take over your life. I know I feel more irritable and emotional, and my husband feels helpless and worried. Makes for a difficult combination!"

Stonewalling:

The fourth toxin is stonewalling. Stonewalling is a very typical response to contempt. You know what happens when people stonewall? They just withdraw. They just go silent. They just stop responding. Have you seen that in your relationship? They either turn away or act busy in some way, like working on their laptop or looking at their phone or appearing lost in their own thoughts.

Stonewalling results in a psychological flood that prevents people from having a rational discussion. The person is using avoidance tactics or shuts down because they just cannot take anything anymore. Contempt becomes too much of a psychological overload. That's why they stonewall.

So, these are the four toxins in a relationship: criticism, defensiveness, contempt, and stonewalling. What should you do? There is good news.

There are antidotes for these toxins. I'll share some of them. I'll start with stonewalling. If somebody is stonewalling you, the best thing to do at the time is just take some time off—twenty minutes, thirty minutes—just get away from that place. Get away from that location. Go for a walk. Clear your head and then come back to the conversation. If you find that you're criticizing the person and not the situation, tell them "I wish you cared about me or you would ask me how my appointment went." Because oftentimes there is a request behind the criticism when there is defensiveness. If you are defending your stance as a response to criticism, this is when you need to start actively listening. Why is this person criticizing me? Pay some attention. Because even if they're criticizing, if they're blaming you and not the problem, there's a 2 percent truth that something is not working. Take responsibility, at least partially.

I generally recommend that each of you pay attention. Ask your wife or your husband, "How are you doing? How are you feeling?" These may not be questions that we ask, but we should ask them every day. It doesn't matter whether you are going through infertility or not. I'll share a story from one of my clients, who actually asked her husband how he was doing this past Father's Day. They were just driving together, and she asked the simple question, "How are you doing?" Because it was Father's Day.

You know what happened?

The male partner immediately broke down.

She had never seen anything like that. Men go through this too. They just show it differently, and as women, we typically don't pay attention to those signs. Allow your man to be vulnerable.

Women can be vulnerable more easily if they have a safe space, but it's not easy for men to be vulnerable. But allowing your man to be vulnerable will actually bring you closer together. Having that vulnerability in your relationship brings you closer together.

And this is something I share as a tip with the couples I work with. When you are going through hard times, through the sucky part of the journey, and you are in the middle of the process, say this: "Together we will make it through this too." I'll say it again: "Together we will make it through this too."

Saying it out loud like that makes a world of difference— you're actually comforting each other. "No matter what happens, we are both in this together." And do you know what the best antidote for contempt is? Intentional and genuine appreciation for each other. You're always looking at each other sarcastically, right? This hostile humor, the name-calling because you don't want to appreciate each other. You don't show respect for each other. Show some intentional and genuine appreciation. And when there is wrongdoing on either one of your parts, please apologize.

This is one of my favorites. Your infertility journey is not the ONLY thing that's happened in your life. You've had some amazing things happen in your past even though it's sucking right now. Remind yourself of that. Look at the pictures from the best vacation the two of you took, or look at your wedding album. Why did you come together in the first place? Why did you say "I do"? Remind yourself of what made you come together. What made you choose to be each other's partner in the first place? Reminding yourself of all those good memories will really help you appreciate where you are now and how far you have come in your relationship.

Finally, don't be afraid to seek help from a professional like me. A professional coach can offer you a safe space to explore your challenges and give you practical tools and techniques to help you repair and rejuvenate your relationship and make it stronger together, no matter where you are in your journey.

My deep desire for couples is that infertility should not break their relationship. It should not. When I was going through it, I had many hardships in my relationship with my husband. He's an amazing person, but that invisible wall kept going up, and we were having a hard time. I was so close to thinking, "Why am I in this relationship?" My journey taught me that infertility should never be the cause of a separation. As of the writing of this book, my husband and I have been married for nineteen years.

If you can't do it by yourself, seek professional help because a divorce is not worth it. Separation is not worth it. Be intentional about the antidotes if you see any of the four toxins in your relationship.

Break the invisible wall between you and your partner. The workbook activities will definitely help in doing so. Do it together with your partner. Go to the link below to download your copy of the workbook. Once downloaded, please print it out.

**https://pradeepafertilitycoach.com/infertility-can-suck-less-workbook/**

# Chapter 8

# How Can You Support as Family And Friends? And Things You Don't Tell People Going Through Infertility.

The next topic that we are going to be talking about is family and friends. How can we forget our family and friends who are there to help us when we are going through the ups and downs of infertility, many of them with really good intentions?

I want to ask a question right now to all of you reading this. If you're a family member or a friend, have you said something like this? "You should not delay anymore. You need to have kids soon. Time is running out." "Hey, just relax. Drink a glass of wine. It's going to happen." "Don't worry about it. You're young." "What are you worrying about? The technology is there."

If you are somebody who would say things like this to people going through infertility, I want to tell you why certain things shouldn't be said.

So many people, like my OB-GYN, told me to drink a glass of wine—it'll happen. I don't drink wine. And it didn't happen. We say many of these things innocently, and as somebody who has heard it and has seen the light at the end of the tunnel, I can look back and recognize the things that really stung me. I know as family and friends you are showing your support with a good heart and good intentions. But you may not have experienced infertility.

Let me give you some pointers. Don't say things like, "It'll happen. Just relax or drink a glass of wine or go on vacation, it will happen." Or, "You're young, right?" Those are some things you don't want to say to people experiencing infertility. Coming from India, I've heard people talk about doing rituals and certain practices, things like that. And even here in America, I heard everything from eating McDonald's fries from a certain restaurant to using certain essential oils to going and touching a certain stone at a certain time.

There are all these different types of things that people will tell you. I used to be very diligent about many of those things because I was desperate, I would do anything and everything possible. At some point I felt like it was enough. I snapped at one of my very close relatives for saying something like that because I just couldn't handle it anymore. I snapped. That was not fun.

As somebody who was going through that, it had really, really hurt me.

Sometimes people go through secondary infertility, meaning they have a first child, but they are having fertility challenges with their second child. Oftentimes people say something like, "You already have one. Why are you worried about it? Just be happy that you already have one. I have a bunch of kids. Do you want one?"

Or they may say, "Oh, don't worry. You're only in your early forties, I know a lot of people in their forties who are getting pregnant, don't worry, it'll happen." Another one that really, really hurt me was, "It's so hard for me having these many kids." Somebody said that to me when I had just had my fifth IVF failure. I felt so awful, I just wanted to jump into the...well, I just wanted to die. When people say something like that, they really don't understand what's going on in the other person's life. You shouldn't really say things like, "My husband just looks at me, and I get pregnant." Or, "I just go near my husband and sneeze, and I get pregnant."

This may sound funny to many of you, but it is not funny for people going through infertility. They're already trying really hard in any and every way to get pregnant, and it's just not happening. And here's one more: "When God thinks you're ready, you'll have a child." Some of this may resonate with you; you may even have said some of these things. I know people usually say these things with a good heart and good intentions. Most people are not malicious in nature, they just care. But if you haven't gone through infertility, then these types of statements may sound painful. But for me, you can just take a knife and stick it in my heart—that's how it feels every time.

One day I was at my manicurist getting my nails done, and she asked, "Do you have a child?" *Yes, I have a five-*

*year-old and he was adopted*, but I didn't tell her that. She then said, "Oh, you should have more. Your child needs to have other kids to play with, you know, a brother or sister." I just gave her an awkward smile and laughed. But people say some of these things very innocently, not knowing my pain. So please refrain from saying things like this.

You may be thinking, "You just told me a bunch of things I cannot say. What can I say and what can I do? How can I support someone and be there for them?"

- Offer your physical presence. You don't even have to say anything. Just be with them.
- If your loved one is going to a treatment or an appointment, offer to go with them to show your support.
- Even a hug can make things a lot better.
- If you haven't gone through infertility, be open and honest, and tell the person who is going through it that you don't fully understand what they're going through because you haven't experienced it yourself.
- As a friend or family member you can be there as a shoulder to cry on, as a cheerleader, or as a listening ear—somebody with whom they can share their thoughts and feelings without being judged.
- You don't need to offer them a solution.
- You can even accompany them to a self-care activity like yoga or massage or a meeting—any type of self-care activity.

Those are just some of the ways you can support your friends and family. I know you all have a very good heart and good intentions. So, consider some of the things that I've shared on how you can offer support to your friend or loved one.

Oh, and make sure you go to the link below to download your copy of the workbook. Once downloaded, please print it out. Start capturing different ways to support your loved one with infertility moving forward!

**https://pradeepafertilitycoach.com/infertility-can-suck-less-workbook/**

# Chapter 9

# Bringing It All Together And A Positive Affirmation

All right, this is the chapter where we are going to bring it all together. I am going to do a very quick recap here of what we have learned so far. Infertility is a disease, and like my friend said, it is a complex massive problem. It exists, and it exists big time.

It affects men and women equally. The world puts most of the spotlight and emphasis on women, but men are equally affected. That's why I care a lot about supporting men because men are typically a forgotten entity here. Infertility is going to be a sucky journey to some extent with all the treatments, all the procedures, and all the injections and medications. It affected me it physically, emotionally, mentally, and spiritually. And remember that men and women go through this journey and the resulting emotions very differently. The majority of the problem that occurs within couples stems from not understanding what each other is going through. Your husband is going through this differently than you are, and we fail to see that. And vice versa.

With all the tips and techniques that I've shared, our friends and family now understand what types of things they should not say to somebody going through infertility, as well as several ways they can show support.

Last but not least, couples, men, and women who feel empowered during their fertility journey with a professional fertility coach like me have a more positive experience throughout their journey.

Let me ask you something. Now you have read this book, what is your path moving forward? You get to decide how this journey is going to go. Don't just let it happen. You have a choice to not be a victim. And that's the one thing you can control. Nothing else. Your choice. I invite you to take control of your intentions on this journey. Own it and control it, make it the way you want it to be.

Use and channel your energy so that you focus your energy on your treatments.

And how will you show up for your treatments? How will you show up at work, or with your friends, with your family, and with your spouse?

Please don't let this journey own you.

You own it.

And I invite you to be more intentional.

I want to leave you with this affirmation/inspiration.

Download the audio version below for a powerful experience.

https://pradeepafertilitycoach.com/infertility-can-suck-less-workbook/

Let's take some time to bring our attention to the present and to our body.

If you can, gently close your eyes and sit comfortably with your feet on the ground.

If you have anything in your hands, just put them down. You don't have to see anything. Just hear my voice. Take some deep breaths in through your nose and out through your mouth.

Take a couple of deep breaths, and focus your attention on this day, this moment, wherever you are. Just scan your whole body, head to toe. Relax your head, relax your forehead. Relax your eyes, your eyebrows, your nose, your mouth, your lips, your tongue, your teeth, your cheeks, your neck, your ears, your shoulders, your chest, your back, your stomach, your forearms, your upper arms, your palms, your fingers, your nails, your bones, your pelvis, your thighs.

Relax your calves. Relax your knees. Relax your feet. Relax your toes. Relax your toenails. Relax your whole body. Just be present. Right here. Gently breathe.

I choose...to live by choice, not by chance. To make changes, not excuses. To be motivated, not manipulated. To be useful, not used. To excel, not compete. I choose self-esteem, not self pity. I choose to listen to my inner voice, not the random opinions of others.

I choose to live by choice, not by chance, to make changes, not excuses; to be motivated, not manipulated; to be useful, not used; to excel, not to compete. I choose self-esteem, not self-pity. I choose to listen to my inner voice, not the random opinions of others. I choose to be me. I choose to be me.

Go to the link below to download your copy of the workbook. Once downloaded, please print it out. Capture all your takeaways from all chapters.

**https://pradeepafertilitycoach.com/infertility-can-suck-less-workbook/**

# Chapter 10

# Wrap-Up, Useful Resources, And Next Steps

This is the last chapter, where I'll talk about the next steps and references. I am glad that you made it through all the way to the end and I am so glad that we are here for the last chapter together. So, remember the two things that you noted down before you began reading this book, I want you to take your workbook and go back and read those two things.

My question to you is: Did you get answers or clarification on the two things you wrote down? If not, let's talk, and here are the different ways to reach out to me.

You can contact me via email at hello@pradeepafertilitycoach.com; you can also contact me by phone at 952-693-8839 and schedule a free consultation with me. We can talk about anything you learned in this book or about your fertility journey and how I can help you as your coach, if that is something that you desire.

I do have a free ebook on my website. The ebook contains a list of 100 questions to ask during your fertility appointments.

When it comes to dealing with infertility, your first-time visit to a fertility clinic can be thrilling and daunting at the same time. Many don't know what to expect and can often be unprepared for the first visit.

This list will arm you with questions you need to take to your doctor, so you'll have   successful visit and take-home great information that may help you make decisions about your next steps.

Even though the ultimate goal for a fertility clinic and doctor visit is to get pregnant with the prescribed treatments, the fertility journey and treatments themselves can be very complicated. These questions will help you make educated decisions to choose the options that best fit your needs and your finances, as the treatments tend to be very expensive and many times require out-of-pocket payment.

For ease of reading, I divided these questions into different subsections. Each of these sections has a specific purpose that will help you ask pointed questions. This list is not meant to be hard and fast, but a series of helpful guidelines for having a richer conversation with your fertility doctor and clinic.

Pick and choose the questions that are relevant for wherever you are in your journey, and add anything from your own list before your visit.

When I was going to see Dr. Campbell, I really didn't have any questions to ask because I didn't know what to ask.

But through my experience of eleven years with four different doctors, I really know what all the things are that you need to ask, even on your first appointment.

Go to my website, https://pradeepafertilitycoach.com, and download your free ebook. Throughout this book I've mentioned different resources and websites—here are all the resources that I think would really help arm you with information about infertility.

- SART – Society of Assisted Reproductive Technology: https://www.sart.org/
- Resolve – National Infertility Association: https://resolve.org/
- ASRM – American Society of Reproductive Medicine: https://www.asrm.org/
- IHR – Infertility Resources: http://www.ihr.com/infertility/
- Infertility Education for the hearing-challenged: http://www.infertilityeducation.org/deaf-videos/

Thank you so much for reading this book. I sincerely hope it has inspired you to take control and ownership of your infertility. Good luck on your journey!

# Consultation Session Invitation

I hope you have enjoyed reading my book.

This was truly a labor of love, and it was an honor to help in your journey ahead.

In celebration of my first book, I would like to extend a personal invitation to you for a complimentary consulting session.

In the session, all I want to do is find out more about you and your challenges with infertility.

This is not a sales call.

My only intention is to see if and how I can help you.

Due to time constraints, the call must be limited to 30 minutes.

Are you ready to get started?

Click on the link below to set up your complimentary session today.

**https://pradeepafertilitycoach.com/consultation**

# About the Author

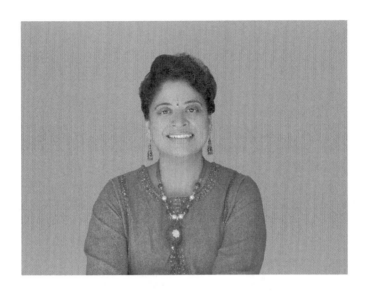

Pradeepa Narayanaswamy is the founder and coach of https://pradeepafertilitycoach.com, which specializes in helping people struggling through infertility challenges. Pradeepa is also an executive and leadership coach supporting various organizations going through agile transformations.

Pradeepa Narayanaswamy is an International Coaching Federation's Professional Certified Coach (PCC) and a Certified Professional Co-Active Coach (CPCC) with over ten years of coaching experience. In the pursuit of starting a family, Pradeepa suffered from a long, lonely, and painful battle with infertility.

Pradeepa's twelve-year struggle with infertility involved having three miscarriages, three IUI failures, and eight back-to-back IVF failures before she was ultimately diagnosed with "unexplained infertility."

After this experience, Pradeepa made it her life's purpose to coach women, men, and couples experiencing their own struggles with infertility. Her mission is to help clients on their infertility journey and to ultimately make the experience "SUCK LESS".

Pradeepa strongly believes that both couples and individuals who feel empowered by fertility coaching have a more positive experience overall when battling with their infertility. Pradeepa is not just talking the talk about infertility, she has walked the walk for a very long time.  pro

Pradeepa is a TEDx speaker and has spoken in various stages nationally and internationally around the topics of infertility, leadership, and coaching. She has also appeared in over forty podcasts and speaks from her heart about various topics surrounding infertility.

Pradeepa calls Dallas, Texas her home now and lives with her husband and her son, Kartik. Pradeepa likes to spend her free time hanging out with her family!

# Acknowledgments

Thank you to God for guidance and protection throughout my life.

Thank YOU, the reader, for investing your time reading this book.

Thank you to my amazing mom, Krishnaveni, for all the years of love and support.

Thank you to my mentor and guide, my late dad, Narayanaswamy, whose vision to write a book inspired me to write this book. I am who I am today because of you!

Thank you to my awesome husband, Sai, and my lovely son Kartik, for your never-ending support and love.

Thank you to Dr. Meera Shah and Dr. Rinku Mehta for writing great forewords for this book.

Thank you to my dear friend Roni Givati for your friendship and support throughout my book writing journey!

Thank you to Tracey Bambrough, Erin Wright, Howard Stanten, Hiba Tanvir, Ellen Trachman and Jennifer White, Farahana Surya Kassam, Paula Bash, Danielle Williams and Justin Williams, Marci Orr, Nimisha Gandhi, Kate Weldon LeBlanc for the lovely testimonials for this book.

Thank you to Christie Stratos for serving as the proofreader of my book. The slicing and dicing as always was very much appreciated, and I could not have gotten this book published without her assistance.

Thank you to my publisher Paul Brodie, who helped me throughout the book writing process and made it easy for me.

Thank you to all my amazing friends whom I have known for more than twenty years. Each of them has made a great impact on my life and inspired me to do the things that matter.

Thank you to all my clients whom I have had the honor to coach over the years. I am very proud of each of you.

# Testimonials

"IVF babble is proud to work alongside Pradeepa in her capacity as a fertility coach. Her blogs and own fertility experience are invaluable to our followers and readers and we wish her every success with her new book. If you have just been diagnosed with an infertility condition, are starting fertility treatment or are nearing the end of your journey, we strongly advise you take some time to research Pradeepa's work—she is a fantastic asset to the fertility community."

**– Tracey Bambrough, Founder—IVF babble**

"It is always inspirational and so touching for me to see someone turn their struggle and pain into an opportunity to help, inspire and make the journey less lonely for others. That is exactly what Pradeepa does. She so sensitively and courageously shares her painful and lonely infertility journey only to make sure it sucks that much less for others. My utmost respect for Pradeepa's courage and passion."

**– Hiba Tanvir, Social Activist, Radio Show Host—Radio Azad**

"Filled with practices you can apply right away, Infertility can SUCK LESS gives women, men, and couples a roadmap to move from stigmatizing shame, silence, and avoidance into empowerment, joy, and freedom. Pradeepa

Narayanaswamy masterfully weaves together vulnerability and self-authority in a way that has readers standing up tall and saying, "YES! I am ready to take my life back." If you're struggling with infertility, give yourself the gift of reading this book and struggle no more."

**– Erin Wright CPCC, PCC and Howard Stanten CPCC, PCC— Vanguard Relationship Coaching**

"Pradeepa's story is an inspiration. She has taken her own years of suffering and harnessed her profound intellectual and professional skills to help others. The tools Pradeepa provides will help those traveling the road of infertility, as well as their loved ones, find a path forward that is less confusing, less painful, and less lonely."

**– Ellen Trachman and Jennifer White, Co-hosts of Fertility Podcast: I Want To Put A Baby In You**

"Pradeepa's personal story is a courageous testimony of the healing and support she brings into the world. Turning her pain into a purpose has not only brought about her own personal healing, but also brings so much healing to her clients. Our experiences are the chapters in our story. The way we choose to share the story will determine the life we create for ourselves, our children and the world around us. Thank you, Pradeepa, for finding light and hope through your experiences and telling a story of hope, love and courage for all. Thank you for being you."

**– Farahana Surya Kassam (Namaskar), Author, Mindfulness & Meditation Coach**

"I had the privilege of speaking with Pradeepa at a family-building conference and heard her philosophy and practices with helping families through the challenging journey of infertility. Pradeepa's message about making infertility SUCK LESS really resonated with me. Her compassionate approach, new and creative ideas for working together as a couple, and ability to tell it like it is was very refreshing for the audience. I am thrilled to see this book published and have high hopes it will help many people!"

**– Paula Bash, Vice President—Technology**


"When my husband and I found ourselves on the crazy, sad, terrifying roller coaster of infertility, it would have been helpful to know a few things for the journey. Of course, we learned all of the medical jargon throughout the years of monthly cycles filled with a seemingly never-ending repeat of hope and despair. But I wish we would have had another voice, outside of the doctor, speaking to some of the ways to navigate life outside of the medical minutiae. Pradeepa's book is filled with help to not only survive but thrive in your marriage, illuminate ways to navigate the emotional toll infertility takes on your heart, and ways to feel supported and loved within your community of family and friends, avoiding the despair of isolation. If you find yourself squarely in the middle of your infertility journey and you're looking for a way for it to suck less, Pradeepa's book will act as your guide along the way."

**– Danielle Williams and Justin Williams, Founders— Legendary Marriage**

"In my time spent with Pradeepa, I have been inspired by her vulnerability to share her struggles with infertility. I am grateful that she is so passionate about this work as no one is talking about this topic so openly and in the manner that Pradeepa is, she is truly motivated to help others. She makes an intentional effort to explore how infertility not only impacts the individual, but rather the entire family system".

**– Marci Orr, M.S., LPC., Clinical Director, Lifeologie Dallas**


"As someone who has lived through fertility struggles and seen struggles of many others over the years, I think your book and course around understanding fertility emotions and coping skills are extremely useful to fertility-seeking folks. The different segments as a woman, as a man and especially as a couple share great illustrations for recognizing these very common fertility emotions. The emphasis on communication is the key to improving relationships as a couple. I recommend this book to everyone going through fertility challenges and take control of your emotions."

**– Nimisha Gandhi, Founder—MyFertilityPal**


"I am grateful to Pradeepa Narayanaswamy for sharing the insights she gained from her own struggles to build their family. Most powerfully, I feel that this book embodies some of the support that she needed when trying to become a parent but sadly did not get. Pradeepa has not only walked the walk but also in many ways is still walking it, by continuing to assist others that are dealing with infertility today. In this book, she highlights the many parts of life that are impacted by family-building challenges, including the relationship between partners. I feel that Pradeepa's practical advice will be well received by those currently trying, as well as their loved ones who aren't sure how to help!"

**– Kate Weldon LeBlanc, Executive Director, Resolve New England**

# Contact Information

Pradeepa can be reached at
Hello@PradeepaFertilityCoach.com

Website: https://PradeepaFertilityCoach.com

Coaching Services:
https://pradeepafertilitycoach.com/coaching-services

Speaking and Keynotes:
https://pradeepafertilitycoach.com/contact-me

Join our Not Your Typical Fertility Support Group
https://www.facebook.com/groups/NotYourTypicalFertility
SupportGroup/

Follow Pradeepa on Instagram
https://www.instagram.com/pradeepafertilitycoach/

Follow Pradeepa on Twitter @NPradeepa
https://twitter.com/NPradeepa

Like Pradeepa's page on Facebook
https://www.facebook.com/PradeepaFertilityCoach/

Connect with Pradeepa on
https://www.linkedin.com/in/pradeepanarayanaswamy/

# Feedback Request

Please leave a review for my book as I would greatly appreciate your feedback.

If for some reason you did not enjoy the book, please contact me at <u>Hello@PradeepaFertilityCoach.com</u> to discuss prior to leaving a review, and please feel free to let me know how the book can be improved. My sincere gratitude to all of you!

Made in the USA
Columbia, SC
31 January 2020

87322393R00054